TRUST YOURSELF

A Personal Yoga Practice Sourcebook

By

Molly Candy Jones

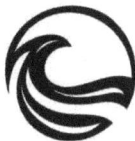

Santosha Press

Trust Yourself
A Personal Yoga Practice Sourcebook

ISBN: 978-0-578-91665-1
Library of Congress Control Number: 2021939294

Printed in the United States of America

For Craig, Katie and Olivia

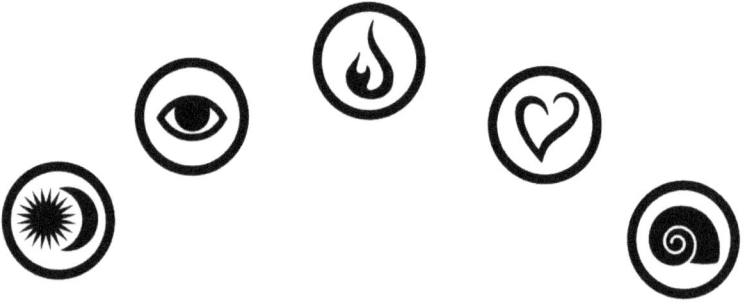

CONTENTS

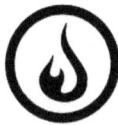

"Practice is the best of all instructors."

∞

PUBLILIUS SYRUS, FIRST CENTURY BC

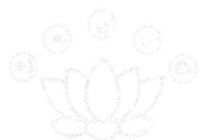

CHAPTER 1

Let's Get Started

If you are settled in to read this book with a nice cup of tea, I hate to tell you this, but you need to get out of your comfy chair, put on your yoga clothes and unroll your mat. First, we practice. You can bring your tea with you, but I'd also like you to bring your favorite yoga props, a pillow, blanket or anything else from your home that will allow you to sit or lie on the floor comfortably for several minutes. We are jumping right in.

Practice: Feel, Then Do

This is an exercise in trusting yourself to know what you need from a self-guided yoga practice.

Sit in a chair or lie on the floor in any way that is comfortable for you and close your eyes. If you find that closing your eyes doesn't feel right, feel free to keep your eyes open. Allow your breath to be what it needs to be. There is no need to change or manipulate your breath. Feel into your body.

Start by feeling your weight sinking into the floor, from the back of your head all the way to your heels if you are lying on the floor; and from the crown of your head down to the bottoms of your feet if you are seated. Can you let your next exhalation make you feel even heavier? Now let your awareness settle on the parts of your body wherever you are connected to the earth. If it's just your feet, focus on your feet. If it's the entire back of your body, spread your awareness to encompass the whole of your back body for a moment.

Where are you more deeply settled and grounded? Where are you sensing a slight lift? Can you allow your next exhalation to connect the more lifted areas of your body into the earth just a bit more? Take a couple of breaths here, simply feeling your connection to the earth.

Begin to scan your body. Start where you are touching the earth and move your awareness up your body. Identify areas that feel a little tight, or a little uncomfortable, or areas where you notice still a slight lifting away from the earth. Maybe a place in the body feels a little cold, while other places in the body feel warm. Can you feel your pulse in some areas, but not in others? The movement of your breath in some places, but not in others? Observe and become more deeply aware of what you are feeling. Can you practice feeling without judgment? The body changes constantly. Every day is different. Feel into the present; into the now of this breath, in this body, in this place.

What shape or movement would feel good to you? Can you connect what you are observing in your body to a shape or movement that will feel just right? Go ahead now and make that shape or begin that movement. How does it feel? After several breaths there, do you want to move on to another shape, another movement? Go ahead. And when you feel like moving back into stillness, into your original position lying on the floor or seated, go back there, close your eyes and allow yourself the time and space to feel the impact, the after-effect, of the shape you created or movement you engaged in.

Consider this first practice your launching pad. If all you ever do is lie on the floor, feel into your body and then act on that information, you will have developed the ability to practice on your own, safely, intelligently and in a way that is deeply nourishing to your body, your mind and your spirit. You are on your way!

Why this book?

I don't have a hard time admitting that I'm lazy when it comes to exercise. I've tried so many different things, including running, swimming, cycling and just about every type of group fitness class out there. I stick with whatever I'm trying for a few weeks, but then inevitably, I'm done. Over it. Except with yoga. Over the past 15 years at least, I have practiced yoga just about every single day. It's rare for me to skip my practice. At this point in my life, my daily yoga practice is as important to me as brushing my teeth. I feel "off" if I don't practice, uncomfortable in my skin. The reason I've been able to practice yoga every day is because most of the time I guide myself through practice. I don't need to rely on others—in person or online—to guide me. And because I know how to do this, my practice is whatever I need it to be on any given day. It's enjoyable and completely flexible, allowing it to fit into my life easily.

This book is the result of countless moments alone on my mat at home asking myself, "What do I do next?" The practice activities you will engage in as you work your way through this book evolved out of my own work on my mat and from workshops I've held on this subject during my years as a yoga instructor in Texas. They are designed to get you quickly to a critical "aha" moment, that transformative place where you know for sure that you can be your own best teacher. You **trust yourself**.

So many of my yogi friends, even experienced yogis and those who are yoga teachers, struggle with practicing on their own on a daily basis. They feel a bit lost and unable to consistently figure out what to do once they are on their mats. I suspect that deep down, they believe the guidance of a teacher, a guru or anyone else who will tell them what to do is necessary for a "real" practice. This suspicion is based on how I used to feel. Does this sound a little like you? If this resonates, even slightly, know that this book will help you trust yourself enough to move through a full and complete, very real, self-guided yoga practice. Once you've made that mental and physical leap, your yoga at home will quickly evolve into a highly personal practice that is flexible enough to fit into your daily schedule and sustainable over your lifetime.

If you love that calm, happy feeling you have after taking a good yoga class from a teacher who seemed to know exactly what you needed that day, learning how to guide yourself through practice at home allows you to have that feeling every day. I'm guessing that if you're reading this book, you recognize that feeling and practice yoga because of it. You don't need to be tied to a yoga studio, class schedule, favorite teacher or take an online class to feel good in your body from your practice. You can practice yoga on your own. You will gain practical information from this book to help you find your way to your mat as often as you need, and to know exactly what to do once you are on it.

Rest assured that you already have enough knowledge to practice some yoga on your own at home if you have taken classes consistently for several months. If you are a more experienced yogi and have never tried practicing on your own, know that you are fully-equipped to guide yourself through a practice. And if you are a yoga instructor, moving to a consistent self-guided practice is the only way to nourish and deepen your yoga, and continue to grow as a teacher.

If You Are New to Yoga

If you have never taken yoga before, or have just a few classes under your belt, there is no need to worry. You can still move slowly and surely to a self-guided home practice after gaining just a little more experience in yoga. I would recommend that first you go to class at a reputable yoga studio for several months. If in-studio classes aren't available to you, the next best step is to find a yoga studio or online platform that offers live streaming classes, so you can build a personal relationship with an experienced yoga teacher. This might be difficult to find, or out of reach financially, so again don't worry. You will be just fine taking recorded yoga classes from a subscription service or YouTube. Try to be consistent and eventually you will have enough knowledge to lead yourself through a short, simple and gentle yoga practice. Be sure to practice with care and plenty of self-love and you will be fine. All of the yoga classes you continue to take, whether in-person or online, will nourish and inform your home yoga practice.

A Caveat

The purpose of this book is not to take the place of an experienced teacher, or in-person yoga classes. Rather, self-guided yoga practice according to the principles in this book is a happy and convenient complement to your relationship with a particular teacher, yoga studio or school, or course of study in Yoga. We all require the eyes, words and care of an experienced yoga teacher. Just yesterday during my practice, I noticed that I dropped my weight-bearing shoulder inward while twisting from a low lunge position. This is something I have done unconsciously for a long time, and while it's not immediately harmful for me, it's definitely not something that is safe for my shoulder when I do it over and over again. If I hadn't gone to class recently and had my lovely, super knowledgeable yoga teacher point this out to me, I never would have realized I do it. Her voice was with me yesterday, guiding me to position my shoulder more safely over my elbow and wrist. In essence, learn how to be your own best teacher through this book, but continue to learn from others. It will keep you safe.

My Home Practice Journey

I grew up around yoga. I was born and raised in Los Angeles and was fortunate to have a mother who was an early adopter of yoga. Throughout my elementary school years in the 1960's, she practiced a couple of days a week with some other moms in my school principal's garage. These were the days of yoga practiced in pink or black ballet leotards, without mats. Definitely the early days. I didn't really consider practicing myself until yoga was offered as part of the physical education requirement at my Massachusetts college. It was the perfect P.E. class for me: we read BKS Iyengar's "Light on Yoga" and lazily tried out various poses that appealed to us during the weekly hour-long class. When I had time, I started taking the bus to Boston to go to yoga class at a studio on Newbury Street. I was hooked. From those years onward, I would dip in and out of yoga practice, depending on whether I had the time or money to go to a studio.

I started mulling the idea that I could practice yoga on my own as a new mom with a baby and a full-time job. At the time, I was working for a small liberal arts college and while I could occasionally take yoga classes at the college during lunchtime or after work, most of the time the demands of my job and my childcare responsibilities didn't allow for yoga. I needed it though, badly. As I raced out of my driveway to work one cold spring morning, I noticed my downstairs neighbor in Warrior Two just inside a large bay window. He was serene, illuminated by sunshine. Just holding a yoga pose. Relaxed and happy. I was a tiny bit stunned. I had practiced yoga for over ten years at the time and it had never occurred to me that I could practice on my own. It seems so strange now, but I'd never thought about it. No one had ever talked about it. Did my neighbor have a book he was using? He obviously wasn't watching a video. How did he know what to do?

Unfortunately, either through busyness or laziness or a little of both, I didn't really pursue the matter, though I thought about it. A lot. I went to class as often as I possibly could, but continued to miss a more consistent yoga practice. Our family grew, my children got older and a bit more independent, and eventually I was able to practice more frequently, though still always in a studio.

—The Ashtanga Year

We moved to Texas, where I started studying Ashtanga yoga, which requires a commitment to a daily practice in a studio with a teacher or at home alone, except on moon days, rest days at the new or full moon. Ashtanga practitioners follow a set sequence of postures, working with a teacher to master the first pose, then the second, and so on, until they advance through an entire Primary series. After mastering the Primary series, they move on to a Second and Third series in the same methodical way. My Ashtanga practice forced me to develop the habit of practicing at home, as I absolutely couldn't make it to class every day with my work and family schedule. It was tough and required a lot of discipline, but once I was able to figure out how to carve out enough time in my busy day and enough physical space to practice, I was good (for a while). I always knew exactly what poses I would be working on at home.

Ashtanga practice is intense. Many days, I was just too tired to give the practice the energy it required. I also suffered through a painful shoulder injury that I believe was from the unrelenting pace of the practice, and the fact that I was practicing the same poses every day, the same way. In addition, I was still completely dependent on someone else telling me what to practice and how to practice. I was following protocol, and it really wasn't working for me. It wasn't sustainable. So, I went back to trying to go to other, non-Ashtanga classes as often as I could, but again, not practicing daily or even as consistently as I needed.

—I Finally Figure It Out

While visiting family in California, I decided to take a very early morning yoga class. Only two other yogis were in class that morning. When the teacher arrived, she sat down next to the window with her coffee cup in hand and said quietly, "Okay, sun salutations." That's it. I waited for her to say something more, as I knew there were several different commonly-taught sun salutations.

Which variation was I supposed to practice? Beyond a few standard sequences of sun salutations, one could say that there are as many different types of sun salutations as there are yoga teachers. The teacher said nothing and sipped her coffee, and then, seeing my confusion, nodded encouragement to me. That's all I got. I had hauled myself to the studio at 6:30 AM and paid $20 for this? Anyway, after a moment or two of awkward standing at the top of my mat, I decided to just begin. The first two salutations were a little disjointed, and I still felt awkward, but as I took deeper breaths and relaxed a bit, I started to trust myself. I found that I knew exactly what to do. I could guide myself, think for myself, choose for myself what I was going to do next. It was a total revelation.

That day, I realized that I knew enough to guide myself through a series of sun salutations and then far beyond that. I didn't need someone to tell me what to do. I didn't need a roadmap or a guide for my practice. I could figure it out on my own.

If I couldn't make it to a yoga studio, I didn't need a book, video, Wi-Fi for streaming classes or series of poses given to me by my teacher to practice. I didn't really even need a mat. I could think for myself, feel into my body and trust myself to move through a yoga practice with skill and intelligence. This book will give you all the tools you need to do the same thing.

My Diary Entries

In every chapter, I've included a selection of brief diary entries I made about my personal yoga practice during the writing of this book. The purpose of these entries is to show you what a real-life home practice looks like, warts and all. My home practice is mostly self-guided, but you will see that some days I take a full yoga class live online. Other days, I'll stream a recorded class for a just few minutes to get me going and then finish on my own, or I'll combine a TRX workout with my yoga practice. Some days are better than others. Some practices are longer and some shorter; some more active, while others are slower and gentler. Also, there are plenty of days where I need to focus on soreness or an injury, or I'm sick. What I want you to see from the diary entries is that my yoga practice is sustainable and consistent because I let it be what it needs to be every day. I'm not looking for perfection. I'm looking for ease, happiness and the nourishment that practicing yoga in this way gives me.

Consider keeping your own practice diary as you make this journey with me. Reading back over some of your entries can be fun, and can give you valuable insight into what works for you and what doesn't work for you. It also can give you a great sense of accomplishment when you see all the yoga you have done.

The Practices

Each chapter begins with a short, self-guided practice designed to give you the tools you will need to ultimately practice yoga independent of a teacher, studio or online service. The practices can serve as complete yoga sessions and they build on each other. Start with the first one and move through each as the book progresses. Spend at least three days repeating a practice before you move onto the next chapter. If a practice is particularly useful or resonates with you more, feel free to stay with it for even longer. In this way, you can be confident that you are adding to the skillset required for self-guided yoga practice. In addition, you can always return to any of these practices later, whenever you are stuck and trying to figure out what to do on your mat on any given day. I return to these basic practices over and over again. They help me find my way back to my mat especially when I've been feeling unmotivated and disconnected from my practice.

We will spend more time on safety in the next chapter, but for now, be sure to listen to your body and treat yourself with kindness, care and love. That is how you will not only begin to look forward to your practice every day, but you will remain safe and free from injury.

DIARY ENTRIES

12/23: Went back to basics today because I felt so unmotivated. Felt into my body, then moved on from there. Lots of backbends, some balancing and twists. A short meditation, then done before I really wanted to be done. More tomorrow.

12/24: Christmas Eve. Did an online class. Focus was on shoulder tension. Ended up tweaking the right side of my neck. It was a beautifully taught class, though halfway through my mind started wandering and the pace didn't feel right for me today. A bit cranky at the end, though this is definitely no fault of the excellent teacher. Back to self-guided tomorrow to fix my neck.

12/25: Christmas Day. Neck is fine, but not a great practice today. Started out okay, though definitely a lack of motivation to even get on my mat. Managed to do about 10 minutes of standing and balancing poses but after that, my practice was full of interruptions from family. Which was fine. It's Christmas. Finally, I gave up.

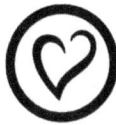

"Go wisely and slowly.
Those who rush stumble
and fall."

WILLIAM SHAKESPEARE

CHAPTER 2

How To Stay Safe

Once again, we are going to jump right into practice.

Practice: Moving Breath by Breath

In my opinion, the only place where we have the ability to fully focus inward and truly coordinate our breath and movement for more than a few seconds at a time is during solitary, self-guided yoga practice. When we are being guided by a yoga teacher, by necessity, part of our focus is outside of us. This impacts our ability to focus on coordination of movement and breath.

Start as you did in the first practice. Lie on your back or sit, and take the time to get comfortable. Close your eyes and inhale deeply, allowing your exhale out through your mouth. Take a couple more of these breaths and let your muscles relax. Then close your mouth and begin to breathe in and out through your nose. Find an easy, comfortable and full breath. Scan your body for tension in your throat, chest, shoulders or anywhere else in your body that may be the result of trying to deepen your breath. Can you allow this tension to dissipate while still staying with your full breath? If not, allow your breath to be a bit less full and again try to release tension that you may feel. It's okay if you are not taking your deepest breath, as long as your breath is comfortable.

Focus now on the moment in time when your inhalation begins and then find where it ends. Where does your exhalation begin and end? Try not to hold between the end of the inhale and the beginning of the exhale, or between the end of the exhale and the beginning of the inhale. Over the course of the next several breaths, stay with this focus. Then let it go.

Come onto your hands and knees on your mat. Align wrists below shoulders and knees below hips. If putting weight into your hands causes discomfort in your wrists, consider elevating your hands by using some yoga blocks on their lowest level. If you don't have blocks, you can place a couple of thick books under your hands to lift them off the floor. If your knees bother you in this position, place a thin, folded blanket under your knees. If being on your hands and knees isn't appropriate for you today, find a comfortable seated position to engage in the following movement.

Begin to move in and out of Cat-Cow Pose, by rounding your spine as you exhale and arching your spine as you inhale. Think about shortening the distance between your sternum and your navel when you round your spine. Gently tuck your chin toward your chest. As you inhale, can you lengthen the distance between your sternum and your navel? As long as it feels good, gently lift your chin skyward as you arch. Avoid swinging your head up and down. Move your head slowly and mindfully.

Close your eyes if you feel comfortable doing so, and continue to move through Cat-Cow, but now go back to your breath. Are you still taking a full and comfortable breath? If not, ease up on the movement a bit until you can once again breathe freely. Slowing down can also help. Once you are inhaling and exhaling easily, start to coordinate the movement of your body to your breath as closely as you can. Try to begin rounding your spine at the moment you begin your exhalation. Finish rounding at the moment you finish your exhalation. Then, begin to arch your spine at the moment you begin your inhalation, finishing the movement as you get to the end of the inhalation. Carefully observe the quality of your breath during each inhalation and exhalation. Notice if your breath changes in any way as you continue to move.

Are you finding that the length of your breath causes you to need to stop moving prematurely? Or are you finding the opposite, with your breath far longer than your full range of movement? Have you needed to slow down your movement to stay within the length of your breath, or speed up?

This practice takes a lot of concentration. Please don't worry if you can't keep this degree of coordination of breath, movement and observation going for very long. Pause when you need to take a break, then begin again. Do a few more rounds and rest in Child's Pose if it is comfortable for you, or in another shape if it is not.

While resting, think of another movement, or even a short, simple vinyasa—two or more poses linked together by the breath—that you'd like to coordinate with your breath in this way. When you are ready, give it a try. Again, start by finding your breath. Then move to observing the moment where your inhalation and exhalation begin and end. Observe the course of your breath in between those moments. Then start to move, coordinating your movement as closely to the breath as you can. Feel free to pause and rest for a moment when you need to. You can always begin again.

After a few rounds, rest in Child's Pose or in a comfortable seated pose, and when you are ready, find your way onto your back to take a few moments in Savasana.

Your Breath is a Key Indicator of Safety

Tuning into your breath on a regular basis and getting to know it better is one of the most important skills you can develop to keep you safe when practicing on your own at home. If you are practicing beyond what is safe, your breath will warn you. Have you noticed how when you are in pain, you have a tendency to tense up and hold your breath? Less scary, have you noticed how your first instinct is to hold your breath when you are wobbling around trying to balance in Tree Pose or some other standing pose?

Unfortunately, if you haven't spent time getting to know your breath, you might not understand its warning messages. The most obvious signs of distress are holding your breath, a ragged, uneven breath or a fast, short breath. If you are overextending yourself, one of these warning signs will usually appear, and it will be patently clear that it is time to slow down significantly or stop whatever you are doing.

Other times, the warning given by your breath will be more subtle. In my own practice, I'll find that I'm breathing "just fine," but if I observe a little more closely, I'm stopping my inhalation or my exhalation prematurely. Sometimes both parts of my breath will be a lot shorter than they could be. Most of the time, I'm getting fairly close to my physical edge when this happens.

I've also noticed that a shallow breath can be related to emotional issues from earlier in the day that continue to bother me while I'm practicing, or that seem to arise out of nowhere. This is not uncommon. Practice can bring emotions to the surface and I will unconsciously resist them by shortening my breath—inhalation and exhalation. I've found that the benefits of my practice are significantly diminished if I do this. I don't get that happy, relaxed post-practice feeling I'm always looking for.

If your breath is sending you a warning, heed its message. You can slow down if you are moving, or you can just stop whatever you are doing and get into Child's Pose or some other comfortable position to regroup for a moment. Feel your breath deeply, relax your body a bit and let your breath tell you when it is safe to continue. And this time, take it a little easier.

Let's take this idea a bit farther. Can you allow "ease" to be your mantra as you practice? Note that ease does not necessarily mean "easy." Can you practice more challenging shapes but still find a sense of ease, peace and steadiness that allows you to take a full and complete breath?

Plank Pose is a good shape to use to experiment with this concept. Can you come into Plank with a sense of purpose, but still maintain a degree of ease? How can you organize your body as you move into Plank so that you remain steady in the shape and breathe? What muscles can relax while you are holding Plank? Maybe just your jaw? Is there anything else you can do to experience greater ease in this shape?

More Safety Tips

- Use an actual yoga mat, not a Pilates or exercise mat. Pilates and exercise mats may slip around on the floor making them unsafe for many yoga poses.

- Check whether your yoga mat sticks to the floor where you plan to practice. If it slides around, consider purchasing a stickier mat or moving your mat to another location in your house where the mat won't budge.

- Consider practicing to 50-65% of your capacity. I know many of you will resist this suggestion. Try to fight your Type A tendencies to ensure that you will be able to practice again tomorrow.

- In standing poses where one foot is toward the front of the mat and the other is toward the back of the mat, the farther apart your feet, the more unstable you will be. Always feel free to shorten the distance between your feet to feel steadier in a shape.

- When feet are parallel, the closer together your feet, the more unstable you may feel. Try placing your feet farther apart to feel steadier.

- Slow movement is generally more safe than rapid movement.

- If you are dealing with an injury, whether acute or chronic, see a medical professional. After you obtain clearance to practice, seek the guidance of a qualified yoga teacher to learn how to modify the poses you choose to practice so that you avoid re-injury or making your current condition worse. Know that sometimes rest is the only way to heal.

- If you are pregnant or have recently had a baby, check with a medical professional before practicing yoga. If you obtain clearance to practice, seek the guidance of a qualified yoga teacher. Pay deep attention to how you feel at all times during your yoga practice, and if a particular shape or movement doesn't feel right to you or comfortable, stop.

DIARY ENTRIES

1/21 Live online class today. Felt great. I knew I needed live instruction to feel a bit better in my body. It worked.

1/22 Felt like I was jamming my practice in today. Definitely not enough time. A few sun salutations did the trick though, to help my back and neck feel so much better. Need to spend more time tomorrow.

1/23 I woke up with every muscle tight. Did a long, soothing practice. Lots of time on the floor and slow sun salutations. Used foam roller at the end. Felt much better.

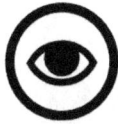

"Peace comes from within.
Do not seek it without."

GAUTAMA BUDDHA

CHAPTER 3

Start Thinking for Yourself

Practice: "Thanks, I'll Take It from Here"

For some of us, it's not easy to transition from being led through practice to guiding ourselves. This practice encourages you to think for yourself during a small chunk of a guided practice.

Wait for a day when you have time to do a recorded yoga class that is at least 60 minutes. Enjoy the class, but 15-20 minutes before the end of the recording, press pause on your device. Try to stop somewhere logical, at the end of a section of the class or at a big transition, for example, when the class moves from standing to seated poses. Then take a few deep breaths in Child's Pose or in a comfortable seated pose if that works better for you.

Now feel into your body and consider. What pose makes the most sense to you after what you've already done? What would feel exactly right to you? Maybe you are tired and your body wants to go straight to Savasana. Then that's the right pose for you. Maybe some other shape comes to mind. Try to completely let go of any preconceived notions of what should come next. What do you want to come next? Do that pose and then move on to another shape after that and another after that if you'd like. When you get stuck, come back into Child's Pose or a comfortable seated pose again to take the time to consider. Don't rush through this pause. Breathe and feel. What comes now? If and when something arises, do that. Keep it simple and when you get to a place where your body (or your schedule) tells you it's time for Savasana, lie on your back, breathe and relax.

Do this practice several times with different recorded classes to get comfortable guiding yourself through a small portion of a class. Once you feel at ease, consider stopping a class even earlier, giving yourself the opportunity to guide yourself through more and more of a practice. Know that eventually, you are freeing yourself completely from needing to be guided by a teacher. You become the teacher.

Self-led Yoga Practice Is Self-Care at its Best

Now that you've had the opportunity to lead yourself through some yoga poses, let's dive a little deeper into the idea of a "personal yoga practice." What is it? For the purposes of this book, personal yoga practice is self-led, self-care on your mat.

Let's break this down. Self-led means that you are your own boss. You determine what you are going to do. Unlike being guided by a teacher in a yoga studio or online class, you determine your own practice for that session, based on what you need. In knowing what you need and acting on it, you are taking care of yourself, engaging in movement, breathing or meditation practices that nourish and heal you.

The idea of self-care gets a lot of play these days in the media. In fact, it's starting to have a slightly negative connotation because it's used so much. As of the writing of this sentence, #selfcare has 22.9 million references on Instagram. However, there's a reason why it has become such a cultural phenomenon. We live in a fast-paced, outwardly-focused world. The idea of slowing down or even stopping to focus inward on what we need in the moment and then choosing to engage in that activity becomes all the more essential to maintaining health, sanity, even survival.

So, why self-directed self-care? Why do you need to do this? You can take care of yourself very well by attending a good yoga class in person or online. However, by self-guiding your practice regularly while continuing to learn from others, your yoga becomes more sustainable. It always adapts to what is going on in your life.

A Self-led Practice is Adaptable

Sometimes, we attend a yoga class that is just right for us. The teacher seems to know exactly what our bodies and minds require that day. Other times though, we attend class with a mild injury or when tired, and what the teacher offers is exactly the opposite of what we need that day. We leave class feeling even more sore or tired. Those are the days when self-guided yoga practice can be a life-saver. If the only class on the evening schedule at your local studio is a powerful flow class and you are dog tired after a long day at work, being able to go home and practice a gentle, more restorative form of yoga is the key to taking good care of yourself.

Even with the huge number of online yoga classes available, sometimes it's almost impossible to find that "just right" yoga class, where the poses, music, pace and intensity of the class are exactly what you need that day. By learning how to break free from being guided, you can lead yourself through a practice that is exactly what you need. You can create a sequence for yourself that is just right.

When you learn to direct your own yoga practice, you can continue to practice no matter what life throws your way. You can practice through:

- Injury
- Illness
- Aging
- Muscle soreness
- Pregnancy and post-baby
- Round the clock care of young children or elderly parents
- Tight finances
- Fatigue
- Vacation or business travel
- Pandemics, hurricanes, power failures or internet outages

Imagine the profound physical, psychological and emotional relief you can find on a daily basis, just through a yoga practice that adapts to you. This relief is yours for the rest of your life once you learn how to practice on your own.

A Self-led Practice Stays with You For Life

Several years ago, I took a workshop with a renowned yoga teacher in her late 70's. During a slow and meditative series of postures, the teacher told us that we were practicing that day just as she does every morning in her personal practice. She described her yoga as now centered on deep listening to her body, with less vigorous activity and more stillness, slow movement, inward focus and meditation. A very different kind of practice than when she was in her youth. This teacher is adapting her practice to her life in an intelligent way. She isn't trying to hold on to a form of practice as it was in her youth. Her practice is sustainable and it is sustaining her throughout her entire life.

A Self-led Practice Allows You to Go Deeper

When you direct your own practice, you can take the time to feel a shape deeply. You can focus on all the various elements at play in a particular pose. How something feels on the physical level; how the breath moves; how prana, chi or life force energy flows while in a shape; where your mind goes. How you actually feel after coming out of a pose and before you move into the next shape.

You also have the opportunity to focus on what interests you. So often we are taught a pose, breath pattern, meditation practice or philosophical concept in yoga class that we never see or hear about again. I've had students ask me to teach something in class because they loved trying it once but never got to practice it again. The beauty of your personal practice is that you can practice whatever interests you any time you like. Every day in fact, until you decide you want to turn to something else.

A Self-led Practice Lets You Have Your Own Experience

Buddhist philosophy asks us to learn truth through direct experience. The Buddha said, "Do not believe anything because it is said by an authority, or if it is said to come from angels, or from gods, or from an inspired source. Believe it only if you have explored it in your own heart and mind and body and found it to be true. Work out your own path, through diligence."

A good teacher is critical to learning yoga and you will have a direct experience of the practice in class. However, only a self-guided yoga practice allows you the time to apply, absorb, fully digest and then quite possibly discard, concepts or teachings you have learned in class or in your reading and study of yoga philosophy.

For example, when lying on your back in a spinal twist, you may have learned from your teacher to use an inhalation as you bring your knees back to center. Every time you do this, you might notice discomfort in your lower back. During your own practice at home, however, you can experiment with exhaling when coming back to center. Does it feel better? Does it feel worse? Maybe you try something else to make coming out of a twist a more pleasant experience. What matters is that you are allowing yourself the time and space to learn what works for you and your body regardless of what your teacher has asked you to do in the past. You are learning your own truth through your own effort. Once you know your own truth, you can apply it in other settings to keep you safe.

Increasingly, there are troubling reports of yoga students who have been physically injured or triggered psychologically or emotionally by teachers adjusting them physically without permission or requiring performance of a shape to an extreme and possibly unsafe degree. So often, teachers ask students to do something in a specific way and don't clearly communicate that the students have options. I saw an interesting discussion of this on social media recently. Some students are reporting being harmed during Savasana when yoga teachers ask for absolute stillness. Savasana may seem simple and safe enough, but to some yogis, mandatory stillness in the pose triggers anxiety, feelings of helplessness, fear and memories of abuse. So many yoga students don't feel empowered to just do what they want, whether it's fidgeting a bit during Savasana, changing position to feel more at ease or leaving class. And teachers don't clearly communicate that students have the freedom to do exactly as they'd like.

In recent years, quite a few yoga teachers worldwide have been found to be sexual predators or serial abusers, or to have engaged in extremely damaging and inappropriate behavior with their students. Unfortunately, some yogis still want to put their faith and healing entirely into the hands of a teacher. These students become vulnerable to abuse.

With all this in mind, the number one message I'd like you to get from this book is to think for yourself. **Trust Yourself**. Own your choices and know that you have agency and independence whenever and wherever you practice. It will keep you safe.

DIARY ENTRIES

3/27 Live streamed a gentle yoga class. Sciatica issues, left side. Seemed to help. Not sure what's going on, but I'm having a very, very hard time practicing on my own. Also, tough yelling myself to do a recorded class. The only thing that seems to work for me right now is live appointments online. Need to mull over reasons why today.

3/29 Super tired, but wanted to go for a more vigorous practice today. Got going but then was nauseated. Ugh. Chose some restorative poses and it did help a lot to ease my queasiness. Just side-lying poses and a gentle fold over a bolster. Oliver wagged his tail with every deep exhalation I took. I think he knew I wasn't feeling well.

4/2 Surya Namaskar-based practice. Kept to simple variations, but increased the number of repetitions. Rolled out back and spine and then done. Felt good.

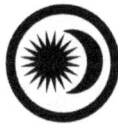

"Who can wait in stillness
while the mud settles?"

LAO-TZU

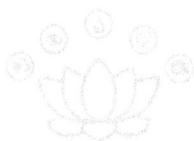

CHAPTER 4

The Roadblocks

Practice: A Simple Vinyasa

A vinyasa is a series of poses that are linked by the breath. The breath is coordinated with the movement into and out of each of the shapes. A sun salutation is a vinyasa. Just as I was asked to do sun salutations in that early morning class in Santa Barbara many years ago, I want you now to practice simple sun salutations on your own, or practice another vinyasa more appropriate to you today.

Sun salutations are something I return to in my personal practice all the time. For me, they are perfect on those days when I just don't feel creative or want to think that much.

If You Are Ready to Go

If you have taken many yoga classes that include sun salutations and know what I'm asking you to do, you are ready. Start by standing at the top of your mat with eyes closed. Take a few deep breaths and as you breathe bring your awareness down to your feet. Can you feel the bottoms of your feet on your mat? Can you now even out the distribution of weight among the base of your big toe, base of your littlest toe and the center of your heel? Root down firmly into the earth through those three points. When you are ready, begin your sun salutation.

You may feel a little awkward at first, and you may have a hard time trying to remember a sequence. Just keep it simple. Go very slowly for the first two or three, taking enough time to figure it out. Then, when you are comfortable, begin to coordinate your movements with your breath. Can you allow the breath to lead you through the sequence of shapes?

Practice as many simple sun salutations as you like. You can even begin to mix some other standing poses or backbends into the mix, if you want. When you are ready, feel free to get as creative as you want. Remember, it's your practice. You can do what you'd like.

If you get stuck wondering what to do next, just go back to your most simple variation of a sun salutation. Know that you can always return to that variation.

When you are finished, take a few breaths in Child's Pose if that shape is comfortable for you, then move to lying on your back in Savasana. Or just move directly to Savasana.

If You Are Stuck Standing at the Top of Your Mat

No worries if you are mystified and have no idea what a sun salutation is, or if you know what a "classic" sun salutation is but don't want to practice those poses today. Many yoga classes and certain styles of yoga don't include sun salutations. Rightly so, as sometimes the sequence of poses isn't appropriate for all people.

I've included two different vinyasas for you to try, one standing and another seated. Take a look at the illustrations and decide which simple vinyasa you'd like to try. While you are working your way through the sequence, be sure to take some deep breaths. Use blocks or any other props you'd like as you move through the shapes. For example, try blocks under your hands during the forward fold and the half lift in the standing vinyasa, or blocks under your hands when you fold forward during the seated vinyasa. Sitting on a folded blanket for the seated vinyasa might make your lower back happier. It's up to you what props you use to support your body and increase your comfort during this practice.

Stay in any of the poses for as many breaths as you'd like. Once you feel more comfortable, begin to try to coordinate your movement with your breath. Don't worry about when to breathe in or breathe out. Just breathe as comfortably as you can and move with your breath to the best of your ability. Whatever vinyasa you choose, once you feel ready, you can add in some other shapes or movements that feel just right for you. Get as creative as you'd like. There is no right or wrong, no correct or incorrect way to practice these. Just breathe, take your time, enjoy and allow yourself to experiment with what feels good and "just right" in the moment. **Trust Yourself**.

When you are finished, take a few breaths in Child's Pose if that shape is comfortable for you, then move to lying on your back in Savasana. Or just move directly to Savasana.

Seated Vinyasa

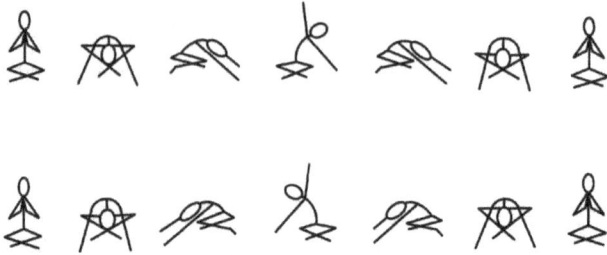

Standing Vinyasa

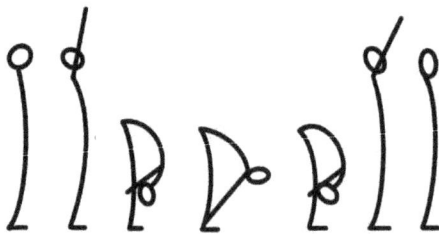

Why Has Home Practice Not Worked for You?

The practices in each of the chapters of this book are moving you slowly and steadily to self-guided yoga practice. However, sometimes it's practicing *at home* that is the primary problem for many yogis. Is this you? Possibly you've tried your local yoga studio's online platform or some YouTube videos. Or you've done a sequence picked up from a book or yoga magazine. Maybe you've even tried to guide yourself through a practice. Somehow, it just doesn't stick.

If you are dying to get back into a yoga studio after attempting to practice yoga at home, know that you are not alone. Yogis have a long list of good reasons why home practice doesn't work for them.

Here are just a few of the roadblocks to practicing at home I've heard from my yogi friends and students:

"Am I doing the poses right?"

"I don't have enough time for a full practice."

"I get so bored."

"Online classes are hit or miss for me. A lot of times they don't give me the kind of class I want."

"There's no privacy in my house."

"My cats (dogs, kids...) won't get off my mat."

"I start noticing the dust bunnies under my sofa and then I can't practice."

"I just can't make myself do it."

"I don't get that great after-class feeling by practicing on my own."

"It's not enough of a workout for me."

Consider some of your own ideas on home practice. Do you identify with a few of the roadblocks listed above, or do you have other reasons why practicing at home hasn't worked for you? Spend some time getting very clear on why practicing at home may have been difficult for you in the past. In addition to mulling it over, feel free to journal on this or even just write a simple list. Clarity on this issue is important. Getting to a place where you can move beyond your own reasons for staying off your mat and toward a consistent home practice is of huge importance to your mental and physical health. Practicing yoga, whether in the studio or at home, is a powerful tool to keep you healthy.

Just in case you need a little reminder, the following are a few evidence-based benefits of your yoga practice:

- Decreases stress by lowering cortisol, the primary stress hormone

- Relieves anxiety

- May reduce inflammation

- Could improve heart health

- Improves quality of life for seniors

- Improves quality of life as an adjunct therapy for some medical conditions including breast cancer

- May fight depression by influencing the production of stress hormones in the body

- Could reduce chronic pain

- Could promote sleep quality

- Improves flexibility and balance

- Could help improve breathing and lung function

- May relieve migraines

- Promotes mindful eating and healthy eating habits

- Can increase strength[1]

The next chapter will help you overcome the most common barriers to practicing at home, and give you the help you need to find your way to your mat daily, weekly or whenever you most need yoga.

DIARY ENTRIES

5/26 Long walk with Oliver first, then TRX, then yoga. Primarily a wind-down, cool-down practice. Twists, neck release, shoulder rolls, lots of time in legs-up-the-wall, plus a couple of different, seated forward folds. Needed this well-rounded day.

5/27 Another of my own practices at the end of a long day. Not sleeping, super tired, and a slow, more restorative practice was in order. Primarily hips, and the only standing poses were a series of three very slow half sun salutations. Rolled out my back on my yoga wheel and felt much, much better afterward.

5/29 Headache today, so I sat on my bolster, closed my eyes and tried to soften around the pain I feel in my head. Then just a soft, easy breathing practice, being sure not to hold at all between my breaths. That's all I could do today. Hopefully, I'll feel better tomorrow.

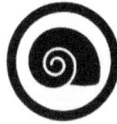

"Work consists of whatever
a body is obliged to do.
Play consists of whatever
a body is not obliged to do."

MARK TWAIN

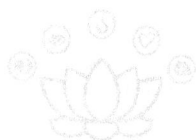

CHAPTER 5

Moving Beyond the Roadblocks

Practice: Pick Five Poses

Have a piece of paper and a pen next to your mat. Lie on your mat on your back. Wiggle around a bit to get comfortable, and then take a few deep cleansing breaths, breathing in through your nose and breathing out through your mouth. With every exhalation, allow yourself to sink more fully into your mat. When you are ready, go back to your natural breath.

Now ask yourself the following question: What five poses do I want to do from this position? If you are newer to yoga, three poses is fine if five seems like too many.

Consider simple shapes or movements that would feel good to your body. It doesn't even need to be yoga per se. A simple twist? Then bridge pose? Then a gentle hug of your knees into your chest, and a few breaths gently rocking from side to side before happy baby? Or a few breaths with legs extended skyward, then happy baby, then knees bent and feet down to slowly rock your legs from side to side moving into a couple of different twists? You can also do the same pose or movement twice or more. Anything goes, as long as the sequence is simple, easy and most important, enjoyable. It seems like there would be no way to forget just five poses, but take the time to write down the sequence of shapes you want to move through. It's refreshing to let go of the need to remember anything or think much. Let your brain relax.

Spend as much time in each pose as you want. That's where writing down the poses ahead of time might help you. Give yourself the opportunity to really take your time, feel a shape deeply and take as many complete breaths as you'd like while in the shapes. Let yourself be fully present, never thinking ahead to the next shape.

Once you've done this practice a few times, consider trying it again but with new shapes and from a different starting position. Two other starting positions that work well for this practice are a comfortable seated position and standing at the top of your mat. Each allows you a wide range of simple poses or movements to practice. Again, give yourself plenty of time to settle and to take some deep cleansing breaths before you consider which poses you will move through.

When you feel comfortable, you can also begin to string the two starting positions and poses together. Start with a series of standing poses, then move to seated. Seated poses practiced before standing poses will work also.

Notice how you feel when you continue to practice by feeling into your body and acting on the information you receive. Does it become a little easier each time you do it? Are you enjoying the process? Do you feel good when you are finished with the shapes you have chosen? Or do you find yourself stuck? Possibly resisting the idea of thinking for yourself? Does it feel like too much work? Just notice, and know that it's all good. You are slowly moving toward thinking for yourself more and more while on your mat, whether in class in a yoga studio, during an online class or leading yourself through a home practice.

Now Let's Break Through Some Roadblocks

If you are like me, the biggest barriers to a great home yoga practice are somehow always related to one or more of the following three issues: enough time in my day for practice, a physical space for practice and motivation.

Time: How Do We Carve Out Enough Time for Yoga Practice?

Not having adequate time to practice is the most frequent reason yogis just can't get on their mats at home. Herein lies the beauty and utility of a personal yoga practice. If you don't have time to get to a studio for a scheduled class, you absolutely do have the time to guide yourself through a practice at home. Again, a personal yoga practice adapts to your life.

The key to having enough time to practice is to let go of your idea of how long a yoga practice should be. If we can change our idea of how long we need to practice, we will find ourselves on our mats more often and the habit of practicing on our own will develop over time.

What Is the Optimal Length of a Yoga Practice?

While you are getting into the habit of practicing on your own, the optimal length of time for a yoga practice is whatever time you have. For real. Once you have fully developed your ability to practice on your own, this can change. For now though, let go of any preconceived notion of how long you need to practice.

Do you have 5 minutes to practice today? Then that's optimal for you. Practice. Get on your mat for 5 minutes. Do you have 15 minutes? Practice. 45 minutes? Unroll your mat and begin.

Inevitably, you will have a day when you literally do not have time to practice. From the moment you roll out of bed to when you close your eyes and go to sleep, no time. That's okay. Know however, that you will most likely have enough time to practice the next day, whether it's for 5 minutes, 30 minutes or a full hour. Can you find 5 minutes most days to practice yoga on your own? Yes, I know you can. With those 5 minutes, you will lay the groundwork for your on-going personal yoga practice.

Avoid "All or Nothing"

Letting go of how long you think a yoga practice should be is key because many of us have an all or nothing approach to things we'd like to do. If we think we need 45 minutes to practice, we will find that we only have 30 minutes that day and then not practice all. If we think we need 20 minutes, we will have 10 minutes free that day and think, well, "I can't practice now. I need 20 minutes, so why even try?" Avoid this trap. If you have 20 minutes to practice, unroll your mat and practice for that amount of time. If you don't have that amount of time, practice for the number of minutes you do have. Most importantly, just practice.

For the purposes of this book, it's far better to practice 10 minutes most days, than 75 minutes once a week. We need to develop the habit of a personal yoga practice. A once-a-week practice will not help you develop the habit. Try to get on your mat as many days a week as you can.

But Aren't Studio Yoga Classes 60 Minutes or Longer?

Yes, absolutely. Most yoga studios schedule classes to run from 60 to 90 minutes. Sixty-minute yoga classes are a fixture at health clubs, and are becoming the norm for many yoga studios in the U.S. because students don't believe they have the time for a longer class. If studios offer 75-to-90-minute classes, fewer students show up. I'm finding that in Europe, specifically the Netherlands where I'm living while writing this book, 90-minute classes are the norm. As an American, it feels like a total luxury to go to a class of this length.

Regardless, we are attempting to break through the barriers you may have to practicing on your own. By believing that you must practice for 60 minutes or longer as you would in a group class, unfortunately you are setting yourself up for failure. Let the 60-minute yoga practices happen later. For now, allow for smaller increments of time to practice so that it's easy to find yourself on your mat more often. You will be setting yourself up for success. I can promise you that the 5 minutes of time you have now will over time magically turn into 10 minutes, then 25, then 40, and before you know it a luxurious 60-minute practice.

Finding Time to Practice. Tips to Set You Up for Success:

• Take your time. Even if you only have 10 minutes, take deep breaths and move mindfully with the pace of your breath.

When we feel like we are short on time, we try to cram as many postures as possible into a practice. The end result is that our time spent on the mat might not be as beneficial and enjoyable to us as it could have been.

- When you practice may dictate what you do during your practice. If you are practicing in the morning, a more energetic sequence of poses might feel right. In the evening, slower and more restorative shapes might help you unwind. These aren't hard and fast rules of course. It's your practice. Do what feels exactly right for you.

- Put your phone in another room if you can. Your phone sitting right next to you on your mat will do nothing to improve the quality of your practice. It can only distract. If you have only a few moments to practice, you don't want to spend it looking at your phone.

- Use a timer. That said, using the timer on your phone when you have a limited amount of time can be very helpful. You won't need to keep checking during your practice to make sure you finish on time. Depending on how long you can practice, consider setting the timer a few minutes early, so you have time for Savasana or meditation to close out your practice. This will allow you to transition more smoothly off your mat and into your day. Just be sure to turn your phone over so you aren't looking at it the whole practice. Or place your phone elsewhere in the room where you can hear the alarm, but not see it.

- Find your best time to practice. You will notice pretty quickly that certain times of the day seem to work better than others.

For many years, I practiced after my children went to sleep. It wasn't ideal, but it was the only time I had to myself. When my kids were older, late afternoon practices were my norm. Recently, dividing my practice into two parts allows me a full practice when time is short. I do a meditation or breathing practice in the morning and asana practice in the afternoon or evening. The meditation and breathing sets me up for a really good day, and the physical practice helps me unwind later on.

- Whatever you find is the best time to practice, don't hold onto it too tightly. Having a more flexible perspective on your practice time will help you find your way to your mat when the time that you were counting on slips away. Again, find 5 minutes to get on your mat. Take some deep breaths and move mindfully. Even in your pajamas at 11:00 PM. You'll sleep better.

- Ask for the time. Sometimes, you need to ask your partner, children or roommates to give you the time to practice. If you assure them that you will be a happier (nicer...) person afterward, I guarantee that they will grant you a little time for yoga.

- Building a habit is easier if everything related to the habit is pleasant. For this reason, I've found that adages like, "If you don't have enough time, turn off the TV," don't really work. You will hear this said about the time you spend on social media too. Turning away from media in an attempt to have more time on your mat might feel restrictive to you. It may feel like a diet, a media diet, and diets don't work. Anything unpleasant or restrictive related to your home yoga practice will not help you develop a positive habit.

Physical Space. How Do You Find a Good Place to Practice?

To me, the ideal place to practice yoga is a quiet room where I can shut the door and be entirely alone. Especially if I am guiding myself through a practice, I need privacy and uninterrupted quiet time to focus inward. I don't have a private yoga room in my house right now, and neither do most yogis who want to practice at home. This is definitely a significant issue, especially for those of us living with big families or lots of roommates, college students in tiny dorm rooms or parents with little kids who need constant focus and attention.

If you don't have a dedicated place for yoga, don't worry, you will be able to practice. Here are some ideas you can try:

- Think once again about time. Can you try to find a time to practice where you might get some privacy in one or more spaces in your house? Depending on the time of day, I practice in an open room in the middle of my house or I practice in my bedroom. Each room works best at a different time of day. The bedroom is the best choice during the day when my family is awake, talking and moving around the house. I can usually get in an uninterrupted hour or so there. I move my practice to the bigger space in the middle of the house when everyone is out of the house or late at night.

- Even if it doesn't appeal to you, consider practicing in a bathroom, a large closet, the garage or even the kitchen. Be open to the idea that you might need to practice somewhere that isn't ideal. The space might be thickly carpeted (not great...), a little too small, messy and not at all picturesque.

Know that as long as you have clean air to breathe and just enough space, you will be okay.

- For enhanced stability, practicing on wood, laminate or tile flooring is preferable to carpet. A lot of us won't have a choice and will need to practice on carpet though. If that's you, consider investing in a heavy duty, professional grade yoga mat discussed more fully below. It will provide more stability on carpet than a thinner, lighter mat.

- Consider practicing outdoors if you live someplace with a mild climate, and if you don't, practice outside on days with good weather. A patio, grassy backyard or larger balcony can all be very nice spaces to practice.

- Know that privacy, while optimal, isn't necessary. It can feel a bit awkward to practice yoga with other people walking through your space or hanging out in the same room. Can you get over that awkwardness somehow? Try to get on your mat, turn your focus inward and just do it. Think also about ways you can adapt your practice when others are around you so you don't feel quite so awkward. Perhaps a more active, vinyasa-based practice is easier when your roommate is hanging out listening to music in your dorm room. Maybe a slower, more contemplative or restorative practice is in order when that same roommate is studying.

- Prepare for Monkey Mind. Monkey Mind is Buddhist shorthand for how our minds come up with near-constant items that keep us from focusing. It is the thoughts that prevent us from getting on our mats. Monkey Mind includes a wide range of thoughts, but most common are thoughts about household tasks we feel we must do before we can practice—make the bed, do dishes, fold laundry, reorganize our underwear drawer. Sometimes these tasks will take up our entire practice time for the day. Can you set aside thoughts like this, unroll your mat and begin your practice? It takes a bit of determination, but you will be able to do it as long as you know Monkey Mind happens and are prepared.

- Gather together your mat, yoga props and everything that makes you comfortable during practice. Put them in a large tote or a basket with handles, so you have everything you need ready to go. You can take the basket with you to wherever you've chosen to practice that day. In addition to your mat, consider props that are lightweight and can be easily carried in a basket: foam yoga blocks, a yoga belt or strap, a pair of cozy socks and a lightweight blanket or sweatshirt for Savasana and maybe even a bottle of your favorite essential oil.

How to Create a Dedicated Place for Yoga in Your House

If you've got a little extra room in your house, you can carve out a place just for you and your practice. This may allow you to have more privacy, and it's nice to gather all of your yoga things together and keep them in one location. Creating a yoga space is also a good way to commit to your practice and honor the place it holds in your life. Practicing in the same spot every day will help you develop awareness of the differences you may find in your body, your mind and your spirit from day to day. You become very aware that every day is different, and every practice is different. [2]

Some yogis have built a yoga room from scratch during the design of their house, while others have converted a home office, dining room, extra bedroom or garage into a yoga space. Many of us have just commandeered a corner of our bedroom or another shared living space for yoga, and that is enough. The cost of your yoga space can range from spending nothing but your own thought and energy to many thousands of dollars. The sky really is the limit, if you've got the means. You will find a huge range of ideas, inspiration and tons of photos of yoga spaces online and in architecture and design publications. However, know that you can create a peaceful, functional place for yoga just by taking the time to clear out an area in your house, re-arrange or organize what's left in the space, and then bring in your mat, props and anything else you'd like for your practice.

Options for Yoga Props

As with the physical space, you can spend nothing at all on yoga props or go all in and purchase a wide range of items to make yourself comfortable. Know that all of the items listed below are just options. They are not necessary to practice. Even the yoga mat itself. You can practice using a hand towel, if that's all you have. We will play with this idea in a later chapter on practicing yoga while traveling.

• A heavy duty, professional grade natural rubber yoga mat is a great option for practicing at home. While pricey and usually too heavy to haul around to yoga studios, these mats last forever and provide a stable, sticky surface for your practice. Be sure to avoid mats that have a strong rubber smell, a slick surface and feel like foam when you press down on them.

Unfortunately, in my experience that rubber smell never goes away. In addition, slipping hands in Downward-facing Dog or sinking, wobbly feet during balancing poses will leave you frustrated and out looking for a new mat in no time.

- Two blocks, in cork, wood or foam. If you aren't going to be constantly moving your props around the house, I would recommend heavier cork blocks. They are a pricier option, but are comfortable for your hands while being extremely stable and supportive.

- Yoga strap. Look for sturdy webbed material with an easy-to-use metal D ring.

- One or more yoga blankets to fold, roll or stack in ways that will support your poses, or to pull over you during Savasana. Look for a tightly woven fabric in natural cotton. Note that you may need to wash and dry them a few times before using to keep lint from being all over your clothes after you are done practicing.

- A bolster. Yoga bolsters come in various shapes and sizes. Most are roughly rectangular in shape, but have various degrees of height. Consider how you might use yours before you make your choice. For example, if you find that it's difficult to sit cross-legged on the floor with an elongated spine, look for a bolster with a little extra height, so that you can sit comfortably on it in seated poses or meditation. That extra bit of elevation will allow your spine to gently lengthen and your knees to relax a little more comfortably toward the floor (consider also placing your blocks under your knees.) A bolster with more height is also a great option for those of us who develop discomfort in our lower backs when lying in Savasana. Many yogis find that they can relax far more when the bolster is placed under their knees. Look for a bolster made with a soft, sturdy fabric.

• If you want a few other useful items for your yoga room, consider foam rollers of various diameters, a yoga wheel, a foam wedge or foam pads for knees, or a simple fold-up chair. There are multiple uses for each of these items during practice, and ideas and instructions on how to use them can be found online and in print.

Motivation. How Do I Get Myself on My Mat?

With time and space for yoga figured out, you are almost completely set-up for success. We need now to make yoga practice a habit. The definition of habit is, "a settled or regular tendency or practice, especially one that is hard to give up." How can we make your personal yoga practice something that is hard to give up?

We see 21-day programs related to health in books and online because 21 days is thought by many to be the right amount of time to develop a positive habit. Diets, detoxes, yoga challenges and many other health-related programs all seem to run 21 days. I've participated in many of them and I can tell you, for me, and I'm assuming a lot of us, 21 days does not necessarily make a habit. I will give up coffee for 21 days and on the 22nd day enjoy my coffee even more because I've been missing it so much. The same goes for sugar and alcohol.

Habits are formed when the behavior is enjoyable. For example, it's incredibly easy to get in the habit of having a glass of wine in the evening or chocolate mid-afternoon. On the other hand, it's virtually impossible to make a habit out of something you dislike. So, let's try to make your yoga practice a habit by allowing it to be as fun as possible, a pleasure instead of a duty.

The following are some principles I've used in my own yoga practice to keep it as happy and enjoyable as possible. They will work for you:

- Start by shifting your internal dialogue. The words you say to yourself are powerful. When you support yourself through positive self-talk, you become emotionally invested in the new routines and habits you are establishing. So with this in mind, try to avoid the word "should" with regard to your yoga practice. Can you shift from "I should practice yoga today" to "I want to practice yoga today"? It seems like such a simple change, but it really works.[3]

  In fact, try to avoid applying any "shoulds" at all to your practice, at least until you've formed a firm habit. "I should practice handstands." "I should work on my core." "I should spend an hour doing sun salutations because I ate that giant piece of cake last night." Anything that feels like a duty or obligation is going to wreak havoc on your ability to create a habit. Can you allow your practice to always be a "want"? Play rather than duty? Fun rather than work?

- Avoid yoga rules you might have heard. The same reasoning applies to any rules you believe you must apply to your practice. Rules are how things should be done, and we are avoiding anything like that, right? Over the next few weeks or months as you work to establish a personal yoga practice, I'd avoid yoga rules completely if they confuse you or interfere with the fun of your practice.

This avoidance of rules includes sequencing requirements, or the order of poses in your practice. Let me give you an example. "I heard Molly say that I need to always practice Fish Pose after Shoulderstand. But my neck hurts today, so Fish is out. Can I still practice Shoulderstand? It would feel so good." Don't worry about any of that. Just do what feels right. **Trust Yourself**. And know that nothing terrible will happen to you if you don't practice Fish after Shoulderstand, I promise.

How to properly sequence poses is something you can learn later, if it's not already something you've learned from practicing yoga for a while. You can study sequencing in books or take workshops to learn this skill. However, the one sequencing matter that I would suggest you consider involves more common sense than knowledge. I would avoid poses that are physically challenging to you or involve deep stretching at the beginning of your practice. Wait until you are warmed up. In addition, I'd avoid them completely if you only have time for a short 5–10-minute practice because most of us have bodies that require a little more of a warm up to safely practice more challenging poses.

There are many, many rules in yoga that are accepted without question by practitioners. I don't think that's a good thing. It definitely can take the fun out of practicing on your own at home. Know that over the long term, you can challenge yourself to take a closer look at yoga rules you encounter, and research a bit to find out why they exist. Then test them in your own body to see if they make sense to you. This pursuit can be a wonderful focus of your self-guided yoga practice. For now, though, no rules.

- Choose only poses you enjoy until the habit is established. Ignore the adage, "The poses you don't like to practice are the ones you need the most." This is critical if your object is to make your time on your mat as enjoyable as possible.

- Don't expect your self-guided, personal practice to be like, or feel like, a taught yoga class. You don't need a complete practice to benefit from yoga. If you want to drink a big glass of wine and get into a restorative pose, that's your practice for that day. Listen to hip hop music and practice sun salutations for an hour; you've done a beautiful practice. Sit at the edge of a river and be present; that also can be your practice for the day. Your personal yoga practice does not need to be the kind of well-rounded practice you would expect to get at a yoga studio or lengthy online class. Once you've established a firm habit of practicing at home, on the days you have time you can explore a wide range of types of poses, from standing to seated, and include a little meditation and pranayama (yogic practice of breath control) into the mix. You can do a complete yoga practice. For now, though, just do what pleases you, what feels really good. That's all you need to develop the habit over time.

- Remember that Savasana, Child's Pose, restorative poses, meditation and Pranayama practices are all yoga. Sometimes we get into what I call the "workout mindset." We believe that we must work hard and get some good exercise time out of our practice for it to be worthwhile. If you want to work hard on a given day, then go for it. But if you wake up tired, or even just feeling lazy, don't worry about fighting those feelings. Get on your mat, but only do what feels just right to you that day. If you only practice Savasana for 5 minutes that day, consider it a victory. You practiced.

- #yogaeverydamnday. A couple of years ago, this expression was all over Instagram and on t-shirts in just about every yoga studio in the country. If you are fairly new to yoga, it actually is a good idea to try to practice a little yoga every damn day, especially while you are getting into the habit. If you are a more experienced practitioner and understand how great the practice makes you feel, taking a day or two off will help you find your way back to your mat. If you are like me, you will start to feel so tight and uncomfortable from not practicing that you are itching to get on your mat again. The discomfort you feel in your body on the days you don't practice ends up being the most amazing motivator. You may even find that you have your best practices on the days after you haven't practiced.

- #practicelikenooneiswatching. This is another expression that found its way in recent years onto many yogis' social media feeds and onto t-shirts, but to have this attitude will help you enormously as you develop the habit of a self-guided home yoga practice. Try some silly creative movement. Take some really deep breaths without worrying about how loud you are. Try changing up the way you do your favorite poses. You might discover something interesting. Remember that perfect poses are not required. Make your practice more about breathing, releasing and having fun on your mat.

Everyone who practices in a yoga studio has days when they feel watched by others in class, just as they might be watching what's going on with everyone else in the room. When you practice at home, especially if you can practice with a bit of privacy, no one is watching. It's incredibly liberating to practice when it is up to you to decide what you are doing that day and it doesn't matter at all how the shapes look. You can really hone in on how a shape feels inside. That experience is so important. To paraphrase one of my favorite teachers, yoga poses don't exist outside of real people's bodies. Everyone is different and each shape looks and feels differently from person to person.

- Do less than you want to do. Always leave your mat wanting to do more. If you cut your practice a bit short and keep in mind what you want to practice tomorrow, you might find it easier to get on your mat the next day.

- Give yourself a little reward. Treating yourself to something nice after every practice creates the impetus for more practice the next day. If each day you unroll your mat, practice and then enjoy a small reward, your brain more quickly makes the connection that this behavior is worthwhile. Make yourself a delicious smoothie or watch an episode of your favorite television show after your practice, and see if it doesn't make the habit easier to form.

- Keep a simple practice log. Consider writing a brief line or two in a notebook or on your phone about what you did for your practice that day and how it made you feel. Keep it super short so it's easy to do post-practice and never a chore. If you find yourself not wanting to get on your mat, take a look at what you've written over the past few practices. Hopefully, you had some positive experiences and your notes might just might give you a bit more motivation to unroll your mat. If not, go back over some of the suggestions in this section. Again, you are trying to form a habit. What can you do to make each practice a happy, completely enjoyable experience?

DIARY ENTRIES

6/4 Hips and twist practice. More energy because I slept better, so this was a much better practice than I've been having. I want to practice ustrasana more often. That backbend feels really good.

6/5 Just a Surya Namaskar "keep it simple" practice. Lots of movement and then a long Savasana.

6/6 Knee practice. I need to do some elements of this practice every day for a while to keep my knees happy. They are bothering me a lot.

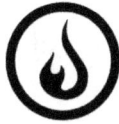

"An ounce of practice is worth more than tons of preaching."

∽⧖∾

MAHATMA GANDHI

CHAPTER 6

Yoga on Your Travels

Practice: "All I need is a small hand towel"

If you don't have room in your luggage for your yoga mat, or you've forgotten to bring it, no worries. You can still practice yoga. You are going to learn how ahead of time, in the comfort of your own home.

Do this practice at least several times before you travel to develop your understanding of how to practice without a lot of yoga stuff. Just about every hotel you will stay in around the world can provide you with a small towel for your practice. This towel is necessary only to keep your hands or your face off a potentially dirty floor as you breathe and move. Can you keep your hands and face off the hotel room floor and still have a satisfactory practice? Absolutely!

Before you begin this practice, please re-read the list of safety tips I've included in Chapter Two. Remember that it is important to stop what you are doing and try something else if you feel unstable or unsafe in any way.

Grab a hand towel and take a comfortable seat on the floor. Drape the towel over your shoulder or across your lap. Try to keep it off the floor until you need it to protect your hands or your face. Close your eyes and take a couple of deep breaths. Feel deeply into your body.

Do you need to adjust your position in order to feel comfortable sitting on the floor? If your lower belly is working hard to hold you up, your lower back feels uncomfortable or if your knees are hiked up toward your armpits, consider folding the towel once or twice and then rolling it up tightly. Place this roll under your seat. Scoot forward a bit so that the roll is under the back part of your buttocks. Can you relax your belly and legs a bit more? Are you more comfortable? If not, consider starting your practice lying on your back with your head on the towel, or even standing. If you've changed your position to lying or standing, pause again to take the time to feel deeply into your body and then wiggle around a bit to get as comfortable as possible. Take a few more deep breaths with eyes closed. Now consider. What do I do next? What is going to feel best to my body in this moment? Are there poses or movements I can do from this position without placing my hands on the floor? Know that if you do need to place hands on the floor, you can always use your towel.

This is another key moment to remember that yoga is far from being just about physical practice, the poses. Where do meditation and pranayama fit into your personal practice? Where might they fit into your practice today?

If you are at a loss for what to do next, for the possible starting positions, I've included below two or three suggestions for basic poses or pose categories and/or vinyasas already introduced to you in Chapter Four. Please use these few ideas merely as a jumping off point, a practice "prompt," rather than a guide for your practice. From your work in the short practices introduced to you in previous chapters, you've already developed your ability to lead yourself through a practice based on what your body, mind and spirit require. Give yourself plenty of time to truly feel your way through this practice. And remember to allow for a healthy amount of time in Savasana. You can do this! **Trust Yourself** to know what to do.

Seated: Seated Vinyasa from Ch. 4, Seated Twists, Side Bending

Lying on Back: Bridge Pose, Reclined Twists, Reclined Pigeon

Standing: Standing Vinyasa from Ch. 4, Tree Pose and other balancing poses

Practicing Yoga When Away from Home Can be Difficult

I've known many dedicated yogis who come back from traveling, whether for pleasure or work, having never once found their way to their mats. Even if they intended to practice, whether in a yoga studio or on their own, somehow vacation or business activities got in the way. That's okay. It happens to all of us. It's happened many times to me, even though I take far fewer clothes, cosmetics and shoes than I should to haul my travel yoga mat and yoga clothes pretty much everywhere I go.

Unfortunately, if I don't practice yoga on a trip, when I get home my body is incredibly sore, my mind fatigued and many times I'm sick. If I take care of myself through daily yoga practice, regardless of my travel schedule, I still may be sore or tired or even sick when I get home, but generally I'm a lot better off and I bounce back from whatever is ailing me far more quickly.

Whether you travel by yourself or with family or friends, yoga on the road can be challenging. You aren't on your regular schedule, so finding the time to practice can be difficult. Depending on where you are staying and with whom, finding a clean, quiet place to practice can be even more difficult. Acknowledge from the get-go that your practice as it usually is will likely be impacted. If you start with that understanding, but then hold the intention to practice when, where and how you can, you are halfway there. In addition, if you apply the principles we have discussed in previous chapters, it will be easier to find yourself on your mat (or bath towel).

What to Bring

While you are learning that you can practice without bringing yoga gear, I recommend bringing the following items on your trip if you have room in your suitcase or carry-on luggage. It just makes your practice time while away from home far easier and more fun.

- Travel Yoga Mat. Thin, foldable travel mats are stable, sticky and easy to carry in a suitcase. You can fold them up to be about the size of a pair of shoes. They are a bit heavy, but worth taking on your trips if you've got space in your luggage. I would suggest buying one in a bright color. I've left quite a few black travel mats in hotel rooms because they blend perfectly into dark carpets.

- If you don't want the weight of a travel mat, consider bringing a large beach towel instead. You will definitely need to adapt your practice to keep from slipping and sliding around.

- Another alternative to a travel mat is Yoga Paws gloves or socks, or a similar product that provides a non-slip grip for your practice.

- Comfortable yoga clothes. While I practice a lot in my pajamas, I find that I have a better practice if I wear actual yoga clothes. A well-fitting pair of yoga pants, tank top or t-shirt somehow give a little lift to my practice, especially if I'm feeling tired or unmotivated.

Finding Time for Yoga and a Place to Practice

Follow some of the tips below to better navigate the challenge of finding time and a space to practice, whether you are traveling with others or alone:

If you are traveling with family and friends:

- Can you find time to practice when others in your room are not around?

If not, try:

- Early morning before anyone else has woken
- Late at night after everyone has gone to sleep
- Nap time if you have small kids who nap or likewise a spouse who likes a good vacation nap or two
- Ask for time alone in the hotel room to practice
- Put on a movie and practice while everyone else is occupied
- Practice with your friends and family. For me, that isn't the most appealing or relaxing option, but for some yogis I know, this is a great vacation activity.

Business Travel

If you travel for work, you may find that time and motivation to practice is an issue, but you have privacy and a place for yoga in your hotel room. Many times, business travel means early morning breakfast meetings, a jam-packed daily schedule and late dinners. If you experience these kinds of days, the desire to practice will be pretty elusive. Continue to apply all the principles on time and motivation discussed in previous chapters, just as you apply them in your practice at home. Most importantly, be sure your practice is simple, soothing, easy and fun.

Best Places to Practice When Traveling

Once you've figured out how to carve out some time for yoga on your trip, find the best place to practice. You might need to get creative. My priority is to find a clean floor somewhere, especially if I haven't brought my travel mat.

Here are some good spots:

- Hallway in your room
- Floor between beds
- Bathroom
- Balcony or patio
- Outside by the hotel pool
- On the beach or golf course
- Hotel gym
- Hotel conference rooms

Where you practice often dictates what you can do. We will cover how to handle practice without a mat on a slippery carpeted, wood or tiled floor below, but it's helpful to consider ahead of time what sort of practice is most appropriate for the place in which you are practicing. For example, a quiet, gentle series of poses and meditation will probably be best when you are practicing in a room where others are sleeping. This same practice might seem entirely out of place in a crowded hotel gym. A more active practice of Sun Salutations and standing and balancing poses might feel right in that kind of space.

If You Are Practicing Without a Mat on a Tile, Wood or Thinly-carpeted Floor

The yoga mat is a fairly recent invention. Over the centuries, yoga has been practiced on dirt, wood or tile floors, or on rugs made of cloth or animal skins. Yoga teacher Angela Farmer developed the first yoga mat after having problems keeping her hands and feet gripping the floor safely while practicing with B.K.S. Iyengar in India in the late 1960's and 1970's. She tried a number of different options under her hands before settling on carpet underlay material. Her father saw a business opportunity in this and became the first retailer of sticky mats for yoga practice. When these mats arrived in the U.S. they were expensive, so in 1990 Sara Chambers established[4] Hugger Mugger to retail a more affordable, sticky yet sturdy mat. From there, sales of yoga mats have grown enormously and continue to grow. In 2018 alone, the global yoga mat market was valued at $11.67 billion. It is projected that the market will reach $17.32 billion by 2025.[5]

If you can't bring a yoga mat on your trip and will be practicing on a slick tile or wood floor, know that yogis have practiced like this for centuries and your practice time away from home is an opportunity to increase your strength. Your muscles need to work harder to keep you stable during Downward-facing Dog, standing poses and vinyasas. Just be very careful and adapt your practice in the ways that follow to be safe:

- Allow the bulk of your practice to stay close to the floor. Consider the many poses you can practice while on your back, on your belly, seated, on your hands and knees or from a kneeling position.

- Keep your breath your primary focus. It will do more to bring you peace and satisfaction than struggling to do poses that are a little iffier under these circumstances.

- Keep the shapes or movements simple. If you are slipping around, stop what you are doing and choose a safer shape or movement.

- Think more about what you can do than what you can't. Just adjusting how you think about the practice will make it more fun. Release any expectations or struggle and enjoy your time.

- Feel free to do a shape or movement more than once if it is working well for you, feels good and is safe.

- Try to keep your palms off the floor and on your towel as much as you can. If you do touch the floor, avoid touching your face. Ideally, I like to use two towels for my practice, a larger one to sit or lie on and a smaller one for my hands.

- Definitely keep your face on the towel if you are on your belly.

- If you want to do some standing poses, be sure to step off your towel. Know that the farther apart your feet are, the more unstable you may be.

- When practicing standing poses, first consider everything you can do from Samasthiti, standing tall with your feet hip-width apart or together. Consider simple balancing poses, sidebends, forward folds or Chair Pose.

- If you feel comfortable, branch out and carefully try to practice some other standing poses or move through a slow vinyasa or two. Again, if you begin to slip or feel unsafe, choose something else to practice.

Yoga Before Flights or Road Trips

If I'm flying, even if I have a very early morning departure, I like to practice a little yoga to feel good throughout the course of my travel day. I've noticed that I'm far more patient, friendly and easygoing during the inevitable frustrations and discomfort of airline travel if I've practiced before going to the airport. Yoga also calms any anxiety I may have about the flight itself. The same applies to long road trips. If I can do just 10-15 minutes of yoga before I leave, my time in the car is far more comfortable and relaxed.

I find that a self-guided practice is definitely most efficient pre-travel. Apply the principles we've discussed in earlier chapters, and don't forget to set a timer if you need to finish your practice at a particular time.

Yoga During Flights or Road Trips

If you are wondering how it could ever be possible to practice yoga on a flight or on a long road trip, expand your idea of what yoga truly is. Remember, Yoga (I'm using the capital "Y" with intention here) is much broader than just asana practice. Pranayama and the preliminary steps to meditation, even meditation itself, can be practiced successfully on a plane or in the car (if you aren't driving, of course).

Whether you are on a flight or in the car, start with some basic breathing. Consider taking a few cleansing breaths, breathing in through your nose and then out through your mouth. Keep it quiet and gentle. Just this will center you and provide calm energy. Then, just as you do at the beginning of every self-guided home practice, relax for a moment and consider: What will feel good to me now, and what is possible in this space and appropriate in this moment?

Get creative and again, think more about what you can actually do rather than what you can't. The following are some ideas:

- If there is room, try a few little twists or fold gently forward toward your legs.

- If there is no room to move at all, do a few shoulder rolls or gentle movement of your head or neck. Round your spine just a little bit more as you exhale, then lengthen your spine as you inhale. Point and flex your feet and draw circles with your toes.

- If you are on a long flight, consider taking a walk toward the back of the plane and if you can, move around a bit or even fold forward, twist or do a gentle standing backbend.

- Before your trip, download an audio progressive relaxation, Yoga Nidra or meditation. These are great resources to have on hand, and will do much to enhance your flight or car ride if you don't have the ability or desire to move much.

Especially on flights, maintain an awareness of the people next to you and around you. You don't want to be that person on the flight. If you don't breathe too loudly or take up too much space, you probably won't alarm your seat mates. Again, you can get creative; just be fully aware and considerate of those around you.

Yoga Practice After Flights or Road Trips

I've found that a grounding practice can really help me recover from that spacey, unfocused feeling I get after a long travel day. Consider starting your practice lying on your back on the floor and move through as many poses or movements that you like from there, but with a focus on feeling your connection to the earth. Allow every breath out to sink your body deeper into the earth.

A gentle back bending practice can really help to relieve the tension that builds up over a long travel day. Most of us spend our time on planes or in the car hunched forward, in near-constant spinal flexion. Consider a practice to gently counter a long day of spinal flexion with baby backbends and other shapes or movements that extend the spine instead.

DIARY ENTRIES

8/17 Lots of anxiety today made it difficult to settle. Did a Surya Namaskar practice with some balancing, but added mild backbends and lots of twists to release tension.

8/18 Knee pain again today, so took a long walk (which made the pain worse ugh) and then did a practice avoiding any stress to my right knee. Followed it with knee exercises from PT.

8/19 Still have knee pain, so worked around it with a gentle practice primarily on my back. Finished with a couple of restorative poses using all my props—bolster, blocks and blankets. Then more knee exercises from PT. Hopefully, I'll feel better tomorrow.

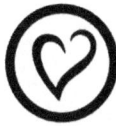

"Why do you not practice what you preach?"

∽∞∽

ST. JEROME

CHAPTER 7

For the Yoga Teacher

Practice: "Wow, I Loved That…"

In this practice you will identify something you learned in yoga class recently and focus your time on your mat on it. Think back to the last few classes you have taken, either in person or online. What did you love? What really interested you? Is it a particular pose? A sequence you liked? A breath pattern? A meditation? An overall theme that you can apply to your practice today? Anything goes.

Since we are getting to the end of our time together, I'm not going to give you much more guidance other than to apply strategies from previous chapters that you've found to be useful. Take your time, breathe deeply and most of all, **Trust Yourself.**

(Safety Note: If you choose to focus on a more difficult or "advanced" pose, be sure to think through carefully, and then include, a significant warm-up like several rounds of Surya Namaskar and some preparatory poses.)

Personal Yoga Practice is an Absolute Must for Yoga Teachers

This is non-negotiable. If you are a yoga teacher, you must develop your ability to practice on your own. A dedicated, sustainable and self-guided home practice has and always will be absolutely critical to your pursuit of excellence as a teacher. When a yoga teacher practices regularly, especially if she can progress to a consistent self-led practice, she will teach with far more authenticity and power. Students feel this. Make no mistake, yoga students know when a teacher really understands what they are talking about. They also know when a teacher is unsure or merely repeating information they have gained from others. If you fully experience the practice on your own and then speak from that direct personal experience, your students' level of trust in you will increase dramatically.

Unfortunately, once a yogi goes through a teacher training program and then commences his teaching career, the first thing to suffer is time for yoga practice. Precious hours on the mat are spent planning classes, working on sequences and practicing the words needed to bring students in and out of each pose. Over and over, I've heard so many new teachers complain that the joy and love for yoga that propelled them to a teaching career is gone just a few months post-graduation from a teacher training. For them, yoga has become about work—very, very hard work. Eventually, the lack of a personal practice shows up in the quality of their teaching.

When you spend time planning beautiful classes for your students, you are working. This time is absolutely necessary. When you teach yoga, you are also working. Teaching is different from taking class, it's not playtime on your mat and it's definitely not about you, the teacher. Teaching is all about your students and holding space for a positive experience for them.

For this reason, you must intentionally carve out time to practice yoga apart from the work of being a yoga teacher. You've got to have time on your mat that isn't work. You need fun. Hours just spent enjoying yoga. Know that you must find this time in order to have longevity in your teaching career. Your longevity is dependent on continually and consistently connecting with the elements of yoga that you love. Why did you decide to become a yoga teacher in the first place? What is it about yoga that you love? Coming face to face with the "why" you practice and teach on a regular, if not daily, basis will sustain you through the inevitable ups and downs of working as a yoga teacher.

Yoga teachers, if what I've said resonates, but it's not quite enough to get you on your mat today, I've listed some other benefits you will gain from a regular personal practice:

Benefits of Personal Practice for Yoga Teachers

- Practice prevents burnout. Teaching yoga is tiring. The more classes you teach a week, the greater the chance you will become fatigued, physically but also mentally. Connecting on a daily basis with why you are teaching yoga and all of the things that you love about yoga will get you through these weeks.

- Practice can soothe, possibly even "fix up" your body after the rigors of teaching. Before I continue, an important caveat: I'm not saying that your personal yoga practice will heal an acute injury. If you are injured, please seek assistance from a medical professional and follow their advice. What I'm saying is that when executed with intelligence and care, your practice might just ease the little aches and pains that sometimes occur after teaching.

Many of us now teach yoga on online platforms. With this format, doing every pose while teaching has for some become a necessity. It's all your students have to look at. You are still required to use clear language to instruct, but now you are demonstrating every single pose in every class you teach online.

If you are still teaching yoga in-person in a studio or one-on-one, hopefully you aren't doing a ton of asana as you are trying to teach. This is a broader subject for another time, but "doing" yoga as a way of leading an in-person class isn't instruction. I've been in many, many studio and gym yoga classes where the yoga teacher stands on her mat in the front of the room facing right or left and guides students through the entire class by doing every single pose. Rarely does the teacher turn to look at her students to see what is going on in the room. Not good.

On the other hand, demonstrating a pose here and there while teaching a class is just part of the job. When you see that students don't understand what you are asking them to do, sometimes only a visual cue will do. Most of us use just one side of our body to demo poses. As a teacher, this is something to become aware of. Also, when demonstrating a more complex pose, we usually haven't had adequate time to warm up or do preparatory poses. The potential for injury in both of these situations is high. If you are teaching 2-3 classes a day, very soon your body is going to start complaining. Inevitably, if you don't listen carefully to its complaints, injury will occur.

Take good care of your body by balancing out the physical impact of teaching with your personal yoga practice. Only a self-guided practice like the one we have been developing over the course of this book can adapt exactly to what is going on in your body on any given day.

- Practice allows you the space and time to feel deeply into what you are doing with your body. You will learn a little more about your physical self every day that you find yourself on your mat. When you can really feel the impact of a pose or a movement on your own body, you begin to truly understand it and your ability to teach that pose or movement is enhanced.

- Self-guided practice fully connects you to your yoga. If I haven't practiced for a few days, or the only practice I've done has been classes led by other teachers, when it is time for me to teach, I feel tongue-tied. Words just don't flow out of my mouth with ease. While my hope is that other teachers don't experience this to the degree I do, I know that my yoga teacher friends definitely have days when clear teaching language is tougher to access. When we've discussed this phenomenon, one thing consistently mentioned is not feeling connected to yoga and that they haven't practiced that much. Lack of practice is causing them to have a tough time "speaking yoga."

- Developing your ability to guide yourself through practice will infuse your teaching with greater creativity and originality. Playing on your mat, trying out ideas, poses, sequences, breath patterns or meditation practices provides fodder for original ideas about the practice that come from you and you alone.

- Time spent on your mat in solitude will allow you to find your own style, way of doing things, voice and perspective. These qualities lead to true authenticity in your role as a teacher. You will find that with consistent personal practice, you can take your seat as a teacher with far more confidence, assuredness and strength. Yoga itself moves to a deeper, more integrated place in your life.

Finding The Time for Personal Practice

How the heck do you find enough time for self-guided personal practice in the midst of all your daily non-yoga responsibilities— and show up for your yoga classes prepared to teach? The following are strategies that have helped me.

- Separate your personal practice time from your work preparing to teach. Your practice, whether self-guided or in yoga class, will nourish your teaching. Allow yourself the space to just practice. Avoid using your own practice time to plan class, go over sequences or think through how to cue.

- If you only have one hour in your day for your own practice and to prepare to teach, divide up that hour appropriately. Newer teachers might need more time to prepare for class. More experienced teachers may have more time to practice. Try to stay completely present during your personal practice, even if you only have 10 minutes and the rest of the time is for planning your class. Setting a timer on your phone can help you by keeping you from checking the clock and worrying about the time. Trust me. That 10 minutes of freedom, breath and movement will support your ability to plan a great class.

- Have a notebook and pen nearby, or use the notes function on your phone. If something occurs to you during your personal practice that you might be able to use while teaching, write it down and then try to forget about it until it is time to prepare for class.

- Be sure to balance your personal practice with continuing to learn from other teachers. Taking a class or two every week from a fellow teacher or attending workshops in person or online go a long way in providing you with new information and learning that will support your practice and teaching. Look at the classes or workshops you take as an important way to feed your own practice. Your self-guided practice time is when you can fully digest and integrate, or discard, what you have learned from others.

Again, using a notebook or the notes function on your phone to jot down ideas, approaches to poses, meditations or anything else you learn during class or workshops is a great way to remember them and bring them to your own mat to work with later. If, however, you plan on using another teacher's material in your own classes—words, expressions, sequences or anything else—be sure to give credit to the teacher. If you know the teacher, it's best to ask permission. This material is proprietary and the result of hard work and original thinking on the part of that teacher. Be sure to give them appropriate credit and appreciation for their work.

DIARY ENTRIES

9/15 Didn't practice yesterday, so my body is really sore. Stayed on the floor for most of the practice—twists, rolling and backbends with the yoga wheel, and forward folds. Just a few simple Sun Salutations, mainly for the folds. Triangle pose just because I knew it would feel good and then back on the floor for more twists and a long Savasana. I feel much better.

9/16 Walked first, then TRX, then yoga. Primarily a stretching and winding-down practice for post-TRX. Focus on twists and neck release, plus forward folds. Needed this well-rounded day.

9/17 Incredible muscle soreness from my "well-rounded day" yesterday. Long, slow and gentle practice to ease my soreness. Used all my props—blocks, straps and especially the bolster—to soften the impact of my practice. Bolster support was awesome for seated twists; under my knees in seated forward folds; under my torso for Locust Pose and then under my knees again for Savasana. I don't think I'll be sore tomorrow after this practice. Fingers crossed.

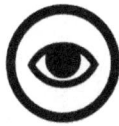

"Think for yourself, or others will think for you without thinking of you."

∽

HENRY DAVID THOREAU

CHAPTER 8

A Strategy for Your Practice

Now that you've worked your way through the previous chapters, it's time to put everything you've learned into action. Today you will practice entirely free from outside guidance, except for the assistance of this overall practice strategy you can refer to whenever you need. I'd suggest that you bookmark this strategy and use it anytime you find yourself at a loss for how to proceed through a practice entirely on your own.

Your Self-guided Practice Strategy

Step One

Lie on your mat with eyes closed and feel deeply into your body. What gentle, simple movements or shapes does your body need right now? Do you feel drawn to a breath or meditation practice? Pick what will feel best, and do that. (Then, if that's all the time you have, lie in Savasana for a few breaths, give yourself a pat on the back and continue your day. If you have more time, move on to the other steps.)

Step Two

Practice your favorite Sun Salutation or simple vinyasa. If you have more time, practice different variations of it or add into the sequences a variety of other poses that might feel good. (Afterward, if your time to practice is almost over, take a few minutes in Savasana and you are done for the day.)

Step Three

Now that you are warmed up, practice a pose, variation, breath pattern or other practice that a teacher offered you in a recent class. Pick something you enjoyed, or were intrigued by and wanted to practice more. It can be challenging or simple, it's up to you.

Step Four

Keep going if you have the time. Think about moving your spine in all directions—forward folds, backbends, twists, side to side.

Step Five

Go back to Step One again. When you are ready, move into Savasana. That's it!

Cheat Sheet for Finding Yourself on Your Mat Again and Again

Just as you might bookmark and refer back to the Self-guided Practice Strategy, the following tips gathered from previous chapters can be referred to anytime you need a little boost back into a regular self-guided yoga practice.

- **Trust Yourself**. You know what is right for you today.

- Make your practice a pleasure, something to really look forward to. Do what will make you happy.

- Avoid an all or nothing approach. You will never think you have the time for a complete practice. If you've got 5 minutes to spare, set a timer and head to your mat.

- Consistency is key to building the habit. Better to practice 10 minutes most days than 2 hours once a week.

- Until your home practice is an established habit, throw out any yoga rules and all "shoulds."

- Try to always leave your mat wanting to do more.

- Whether you have 5 minutes to practice or 60, take your time. Breathe deeply and fully.

- Avoid poses you struggle with or dislike until practicing on your own is a firm habit.

- A little creative movement is fun. Pose perfection is not required.

- Find your best time and place to practice, but don't hold onto them too tightly.

- Remember that Savasana, Child's Pose, meditation and Pranayama are also yoga.

- Put your phone out of sight and reach.

- If you are a yoga teacher, avoid planning classes during your personal practice time. Keep a notebook nearby to jot down thoughts and ideas you want to remember, but then go back to focusing on yourself.

Remember, all you need to enjoy yoga every day for the rest of your life is already within you. **Trust Yourself**.

Good luck on your personal practice journey!

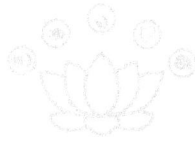

NOTES

[1.] Healthline, 13 Benefits of Yoga, Rachael Link, MS, RD, August 30, 2017

[2.] Sherise Dorf, "A Room of One's Om: Create Space For Home Practice", Yoga Journal, April 5, 2017

[3.] Jill P. Weber, "The Power of Your Internal Dialogue", Psychology Today, July 14, 2017

[4.] Mel Skinner, "Stuck on Yoga: The History of the Yoga Mat", yogalondon.net

[5.] Million Insights, May 19, 2020

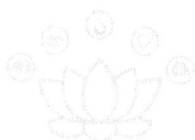

ACKNOWLEDGMENTS

Many thanks and much gratitude to Tiffany Harelik and her amazing team at Spellbound Publishers. Thank you also to my yoga tribe, my "park therapy" sisters, who are ever-positive and supportive, and who knew exactly when to give me the gentle push I needed. Finally, so much love to my husband Craig. Thank you.

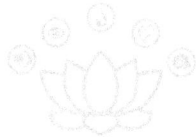

ABOUT THE AUTHOR

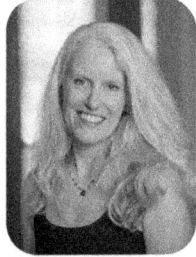

Molly Candy Jones brings over 30 years of yoga practice to "Trust Yourself" and to her workshops for yoga teachers and students on cultivating a personal yoga practice. She started teaching yoga in 2006 and is a Yoga Alliance registered instructor at the E-RYT500 level. Molly lives and teaches yoga in Katy, Texas. For more information, go to www.mollycandyjones.com.

www.ingramcontent.com/pod-product-compliance
Lightning Source LLC
Chambersburg PA
CBHW032150020426
42334CB00016B/1261

*9 7 8 0 5 7 8 9 1 6 6 5 1 *